Organic Homemade Skin & Body Handbook

Step-by-Step Easy Recipes for Glowing Skin and Natural Beauty

Disclaimer and Terms of Use:

Table of Contents

Introduction

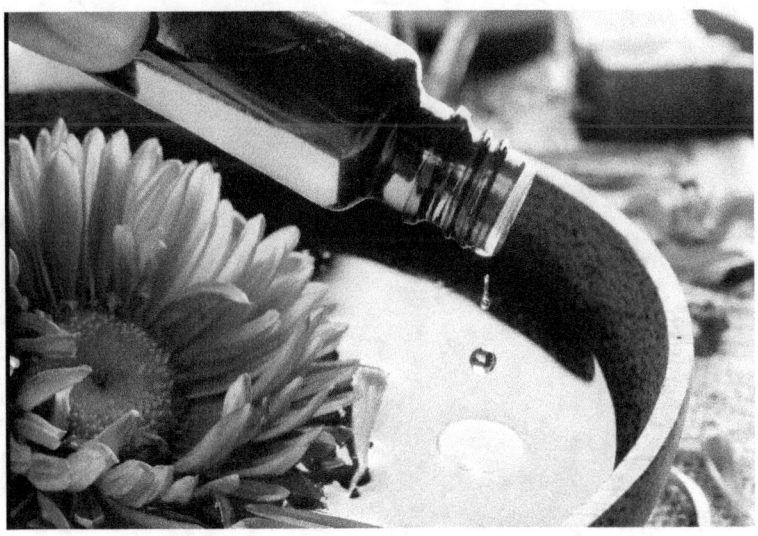

The all-natural and organic craze is sweeping the nation, affecting everything from food to beauty products. Organic beauty products are much better for your skin and body, there is no doubt, but they can often be prohibitively expensive. If you buy your organic beauty products at a boutique or specialty store you may end up paying a small fortune for them. If you want the benefits of organic skin and body products but don't want to pay the premium price, consider making your own at home! Making organic beauty products like bath salts, body butters, and facial scrubs is easier than you might think. If you are ready to give it a try, simply pick a recipe from this book and get started!

Homemade Skin and Body Recipes

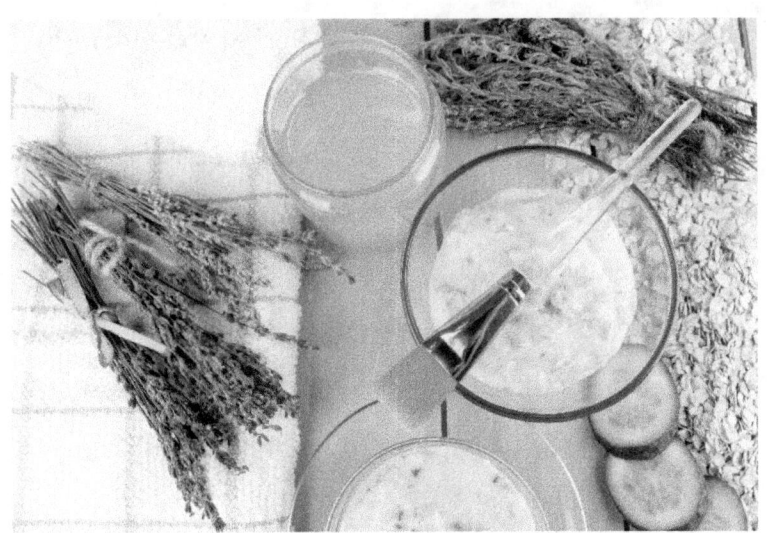

<u>Recipes Included in this Book</u>:

Vanilla Body Butter

Soothing Lavender Bath Salts

Simple Banana Face Mask

Lime Coconut Lip Scrub

Peppermint Rosemary Shampoo

Chamomile Conditioner

Whipped Peppermint Body Lotion

Invigorating Mint Bath Salts

Stress-Relieving Facial Scrub

Spiced Honey Lip Balm

Oatmeal Face Mask

Rose Shea Butter Lotion

Pretty in Pink Conditioner

Refreshing Citrus Bath Salts

Lavender Jasmine Shampoo

Brown Sugar Lip Scrub

Whipped Coconut Oil Body Butter

Lovely Floral Bath Salts

Invigorating Orange Lime Conditioner

Yogurt Facial Mask

Pine Fresh Shampoo

Perky Peppermint Lip Balm

Energy-Boosting Coffee Scrub

Sweet Orange Body Butter

Lemon Facial Mask

Vanilla Body Butter

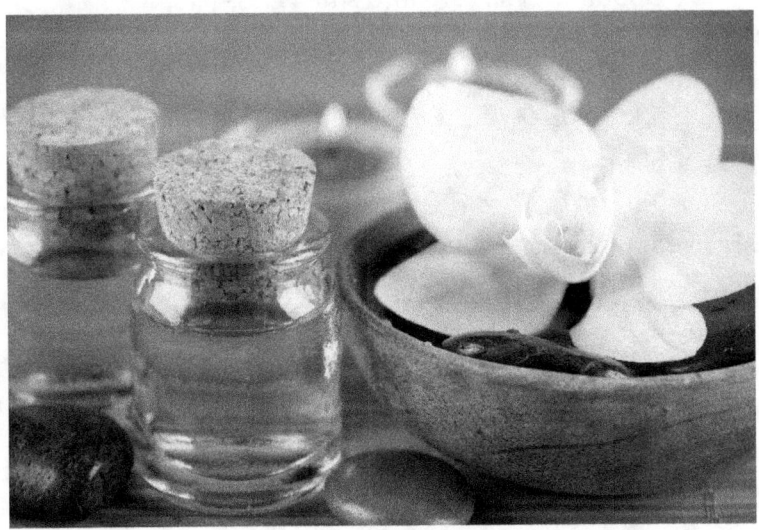

Ingredients:

- 1 cup organic cocoa butter
- ½ cup organic coconut oil
- ½ cup sweet almond oil
- 8 to 12 drops vanilla essential oil

Instructions:

1. Combine the cocoa butter and coconut oil in a double boiler over low heat.
2. Heat the ingredients until melted them remove from heat.
3. Whisk in the sweet almond oil.
4. Allow the mixture to cool to room temperature then stir in the vanilla essential oil.

5. Beat the mixture with a hand mixer on high speed for 6 to 8 minutes until whipped.
6. Spoon the mixture into small glass jars.

Soothing Lavender Bath Salts

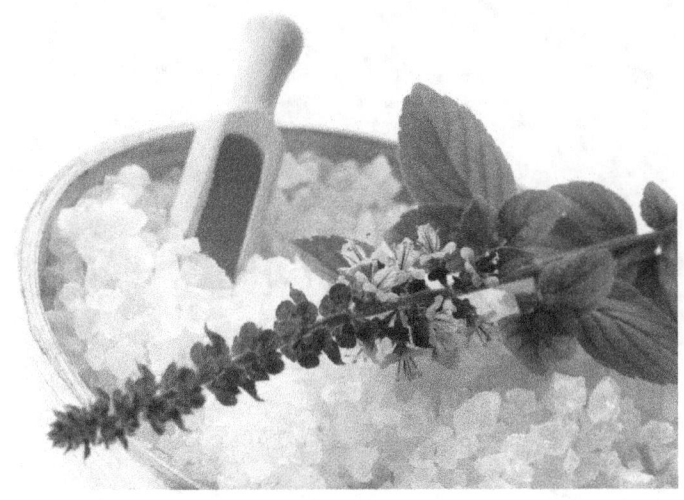

Ingredients:

- 2 cups Himalayan pink salt
- 1 tablespoon sweet almond oil
- 20 drops lavender essential oil

Instructions:

1. Pour the salt into a mixing bowl.
2. Add the sweet almond oil and lavender essential oil.
3. Stir well to combine then pour into glass jars to store.
4. To use the salts, run a hot bath and stir in ¼ to ½ cup of salt while the water is running.
5. Stir the water by hand until the salts are dissolved.
6. Soak for at least 30 minutes then towel dry.

Simple Banana Face Mask

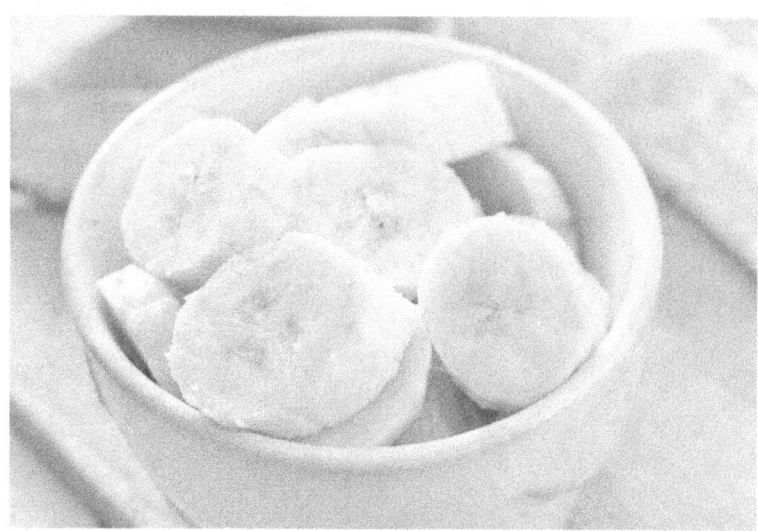

Ingredients:

- 1 medium banana, peeled and chopped
- ¼ cup plain yogurt
- 1 ½ tablespoons raw honey

Instructions:

1. Place the banana in a bowl and mash with a fork.
2. Stir in the yogurt and honey then apply to the skin on your face and neck.
3. Let the mixture sit for 15 to 20 minutes.
4. Rinse with cool water and pat dry.

Lime Coconut Lip Scrub

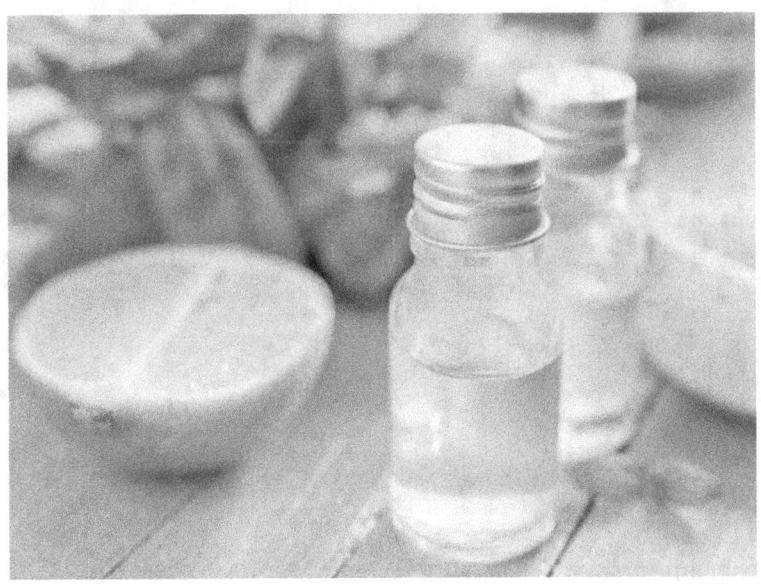

Ingredients:

- ¼ cup organic cane sugar
- 1 ½ teaspoon organic coconut oil
- 1 teaspoon fresh lime juice

Instructions:

1. Stir together the sugar, coconut oil and lime juice in a bowl.
2. Pour the mixture into a small glass jar to store.
3. Apply a small amount of the mixture to damp lips.
4. Scrub the mixture into your lips for 1 minute then rinse with cool water.

Peppermint Rosemary Shampoo

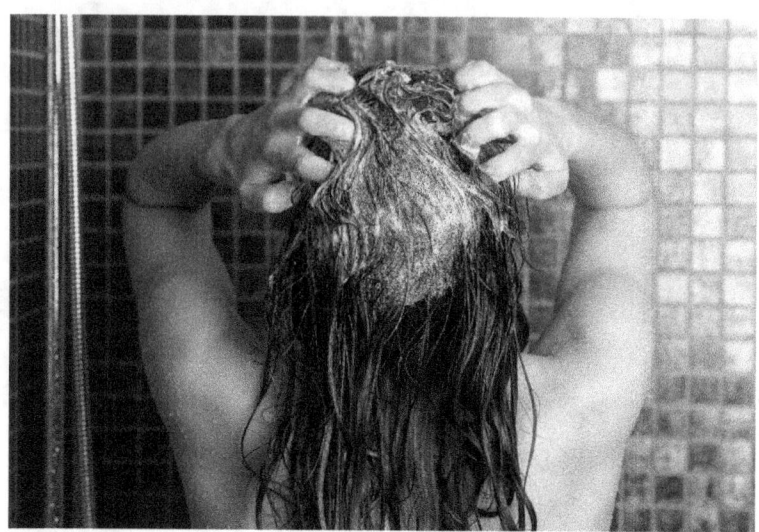

Ingredients:

- ½ cup unscented liquid castile soap
- 12 drops rosemary essential oil
- 4 drops peppermint essential oil
- Filtered water, as needed

Instructions:

1. Combine the liquid soap and essential oils in an empty shampoo bottle.
2. Swirl the ingredients gently to combine.
3. Add enough water to fill the bottle the rest of the way.
4. Shake gently to combine the ingredients.
5. Apply a small amount of shampoo to damp hair and work into a lather.

6. Rinse your hair with warm water then towel dry.

Chamomile Conditioner

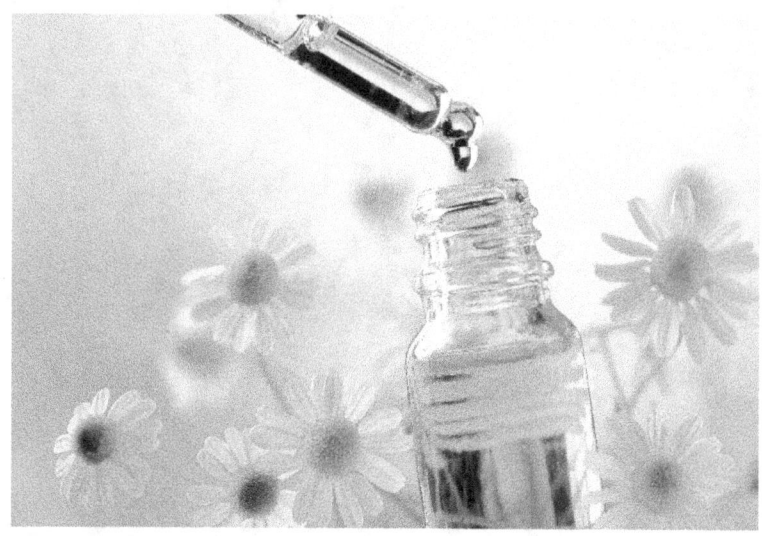

Ingredients:

- 1 cup organic coconut oil
- 1 teaspoon vitamin E oil (2 capsules)
- 1 teaspoon jojoba oil
- 4 to 6 drops chamomile essential oil

Instructions:

1. Combine the coconut oil, vitamin E oil, jojoba oil and essential oil in a bowl.
2. Blend with a hand mixer until thoroughly combined.
3. Apply a small amount of the conditioner to washed hair.
4. Let it set for 3 to 5 minutes then rinse with warm water and pat dry.

Whipped Peppermint Body Lotion

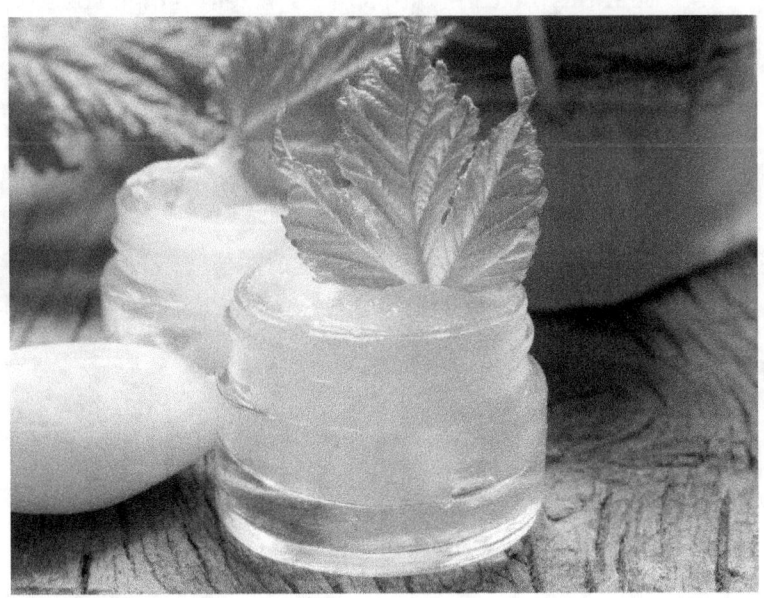

Ingredients:

- ½ cup organic cocoa butter
- ½ cup organic shea butter
- ½ cup organic coconut oil
- ½ cup jojoba oil
- 4 drops peppermint essential oil

Instructions:

1. Combine the cocoa butter, shea butter, and coconut oil in a double boiler over low heat.
2. Heat the ingredients until melted them remove from heat.
3. Whisk in the jojoba oil.

4. Allow the mixture to cool to room temperature then stir in the peppermint essential oil.
5. Beat the mixture with a hand mixer on high speed for 6 to 8 minutes until whipped.
6. Spoon the mixture into small glass jars.

Invigorating Mint Bath Salts

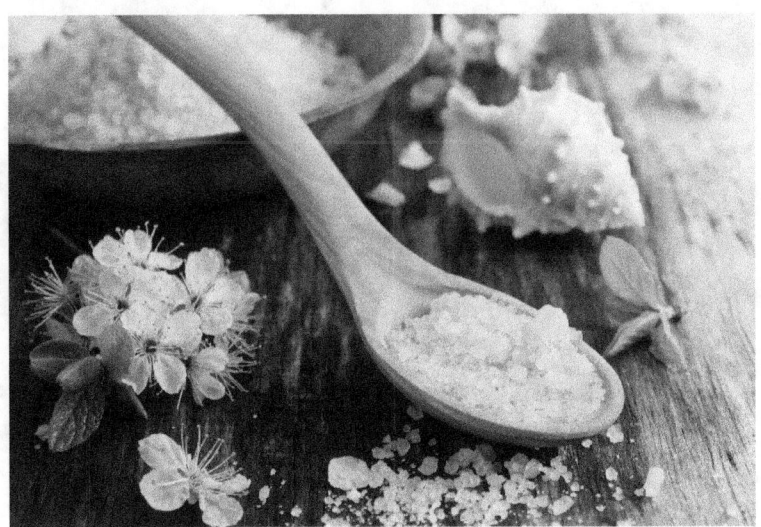

Ingredients:

- 2 cups Himalayan pink salt
- 1 tablespoon jojoba oil
- 12 drops peppermint or spearmint essential oil

Instructions:

1. Pour the salt into a mixing bowl.
2. Add the jojoba oil and mint essential oil.
3. Stir well to combine then pour into glass jars to store.
4. To use the salts, run a hot bath and stir in ¼ to ½ cup of salt while the water is running.
5. Stir the water by hand until the salts are dissolved.
6. Soak for at least 30 minutes then towel dry.

Stress-Relieving Facial Scrub

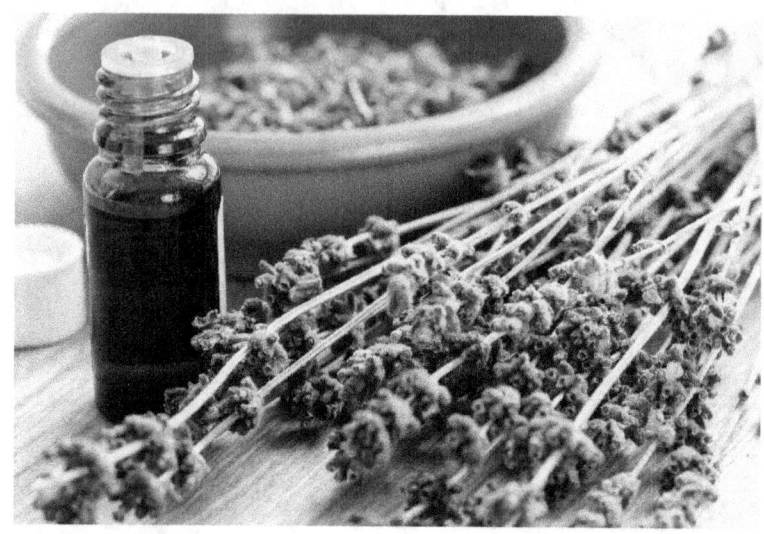

Ingredients:

- 1 cup organic cane sugar, coarse-grain
- ¼ cup organic olive oil
- 2 tablespoons raw honey
- 18 drops lavender essential oil
- 12 drops rosemary essential oil

Instructions:

1. Stir together the cane sugar, olive oil, and honey in a mixing bowl.
2. Add the lavender and rosemary essential oils.
3. Stir well then spoon the mixture into a glass jar.
4. Apply a small amount of the mixture to damp skin.
5. Gently scrub your face with your fingers then rinse with cool water and pat dry.

Spiced Honey Lip Balm

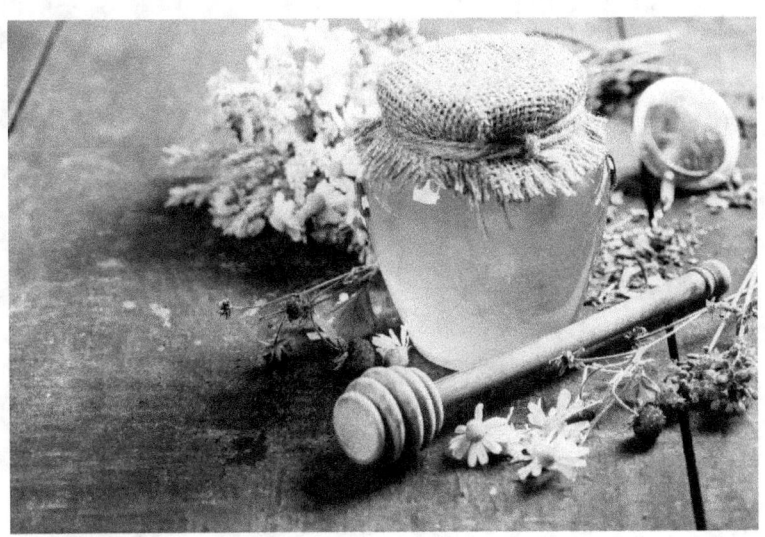

Ingredients:

- 2 tablespoons organic coconut oil
- 1 ½ tablespoons organic cocoa butter
- 1 ½ tablespoons beeswax granules
- 1 teaspoon raw honey
- 1 tablespoon sweet almond oil
- 6 drops cinnamon essential oil
- 2 drops ginger essential oil

Instructions:

1. Combine the coconut oil, cocoa butter, beeswax and honey in a double boiler over low heat.
2. Heat until the ingredients are melted then whisk smooth and remove from heat.
3. Whisk in the sweet almond oil and essential oils.

4. Pour the mixture into empty lip balm tubes and let them rest upright at room temperature until solidified.

Oatmeal Face Mask

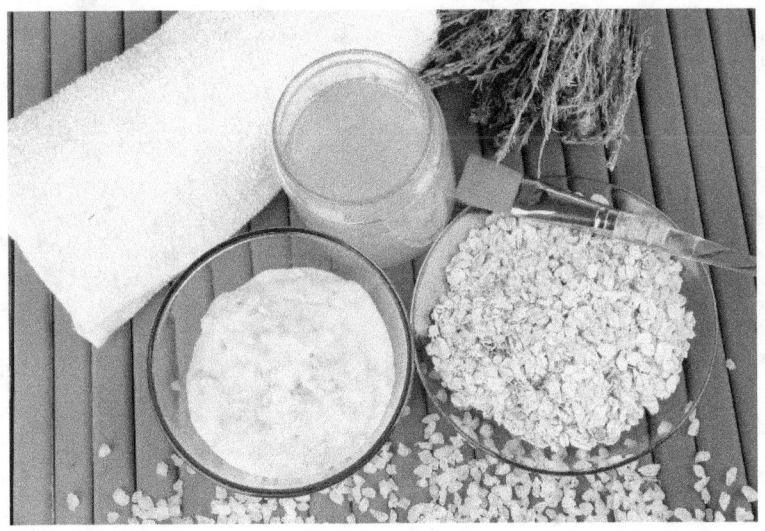

Ingredients:

- 1/3 cup old-fashioned oats
- ½ cup hot water
- 2 tablespoons plain yogurt
- 1 ½ tablespoons raw honey
- 1 egg white

Instructions:

1. Place the oatmeal in a small bowl.
2. Pour the hot water over it and let rest for 3 minutes.
3. Stir in the yogurt, honey and egg white until well combined.
4. Apply the mixture to your face in a thin layer.
5. Let the mixture sit on your skin for 15 minutes.

6. Rinse with warm water then pat dry.

Rose Shea Butter Lotion

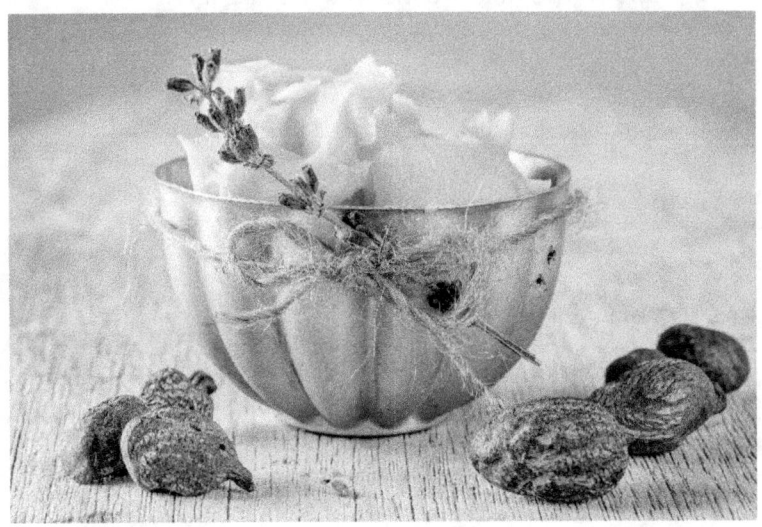

Ingredients:

- 1 cup organic shea butter
- ½ cup organic coconut oil
- ½ cup sweet almond oil
- 12 to 16 drops rose essential oil

Instructions:

1. Combine the shea butter and coconut oil in a double boiler over low heat.
2. Heat the ingredients until melted them remove from heat.
3. Whisk in the sweet almond oil.
4. Allow the mixture to cool to room temperature then stir in the rose essential oil.

5. Beat the mixture with a hand mixer on high speed for 6 to 8 minutes until whipped.
6. Spoon the mixture into small glass jars.

Pretty in Pink Conditioner

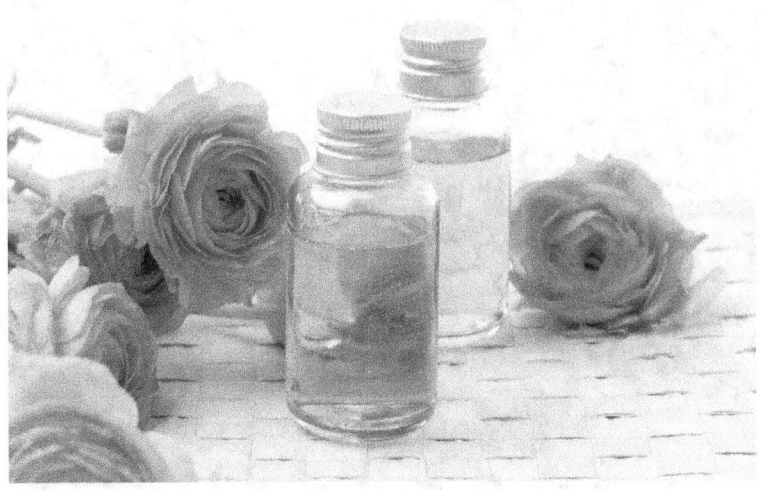

Ingredients:

- 1 cup organic coconut oil
- 1 teaspoon vitamin E oil (2 capsules)
- 1 teaspoon sweet almond oil
- 6 drops rose essential oil

Instructions:

1. Combine the coconut oil, vitamin E oil, sweet almond oil and essential oil in a bowl.
2. Blend with a hand mixer until thoroughly combined.
3. Apply a small amount of the conditioner to washed hair.
4. Let it set for 3 to 5 minutes then rinse with warm water and pat dry.

Refreshing Citrus Bath Salts

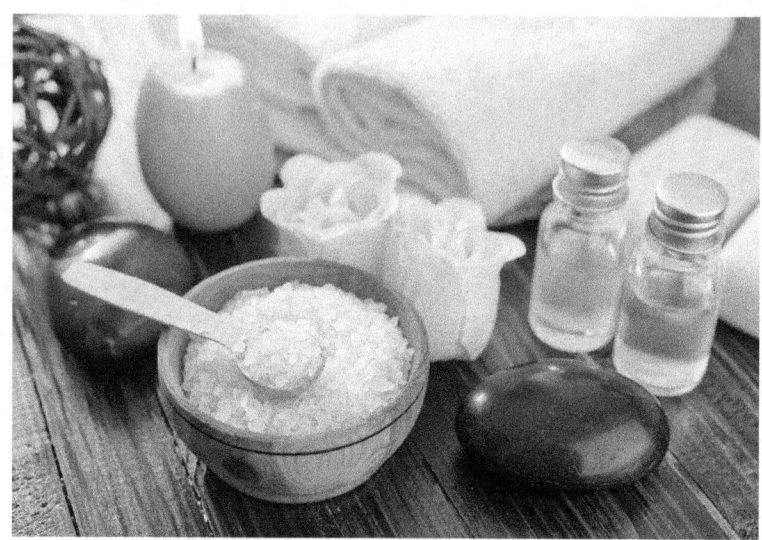

Ingredients:

- 2 cups Himalayan pink salt
- 1 tablespoon sweet almond oil
- 10 drops orange essential oil
- 6 drops lemon essential oil
- 4 drops lime essential oil

Instructions:

1. Pour the salt into a mixing bowl.
2. Add the sweet almond oil and essential oils.
3. Stir well to combine then pour into glass jars to store.
4. To use the salts, run a hot bath and stir in ¼ to ½ cup of salt while the water is running.
5. Stir the water by hand until the salts are dissolved.

6. Soak for at least 30 minutes then towel dry.

Lavender Jasmine Shampoo

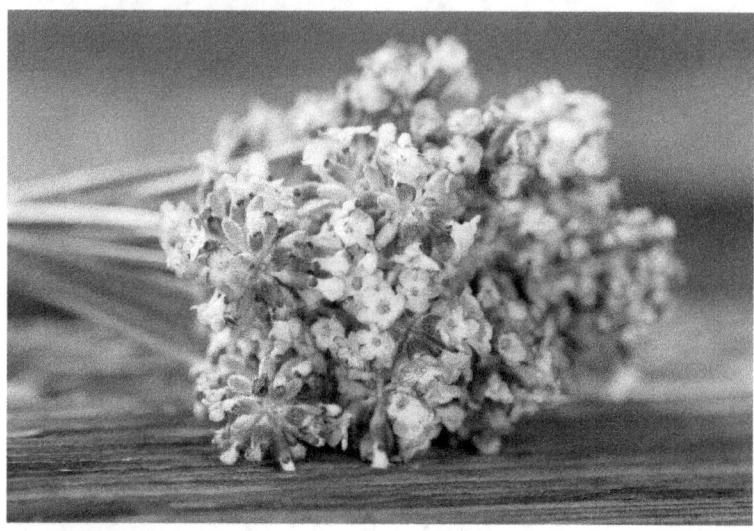

Ingredients:

- ½ cup unscented liquid castile soap
- 12 drops lavender essential oil
- 8 drops jasmine essential oil
- Filtered water, as needed

Instructions:

1. Combine the liquid soap and essential oils in an empty shampoo bottle.
2. Swirl the ingredients gently to combine.
3. Add enough water to fill the bottle the rest of the way.
4. Shake gently to combine the ingredients.
5. Apply a small amount of shampoo to damp hair and work into a lather.

6. Rinse your hair with warm water then towel dry.

Brown Sugar Lip Scrub

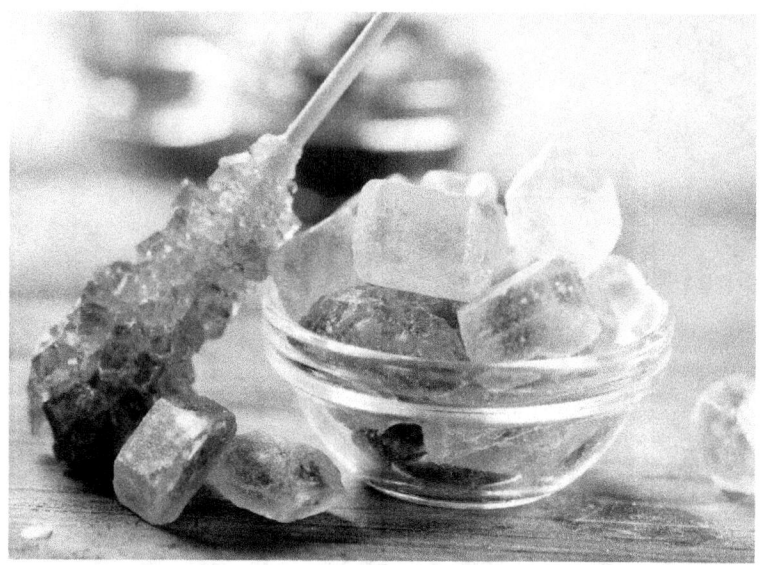

Ingredients:

- ¼ cup organic brown sugar, packed
- 1 teaspoon organic coconut oil
- 1 teaspoon raw honey

Instructions:

1. Stir together the sugar, coconut oil and honey in a bowl.
2. Pour the mixture into a small glass jar to store.
3. Apply a small amount of the mixture to damp lips.
4. Scrub the mixture into your lips for 1 minute then rinse with cool water.

Whipped Coconut Oil Body Butter

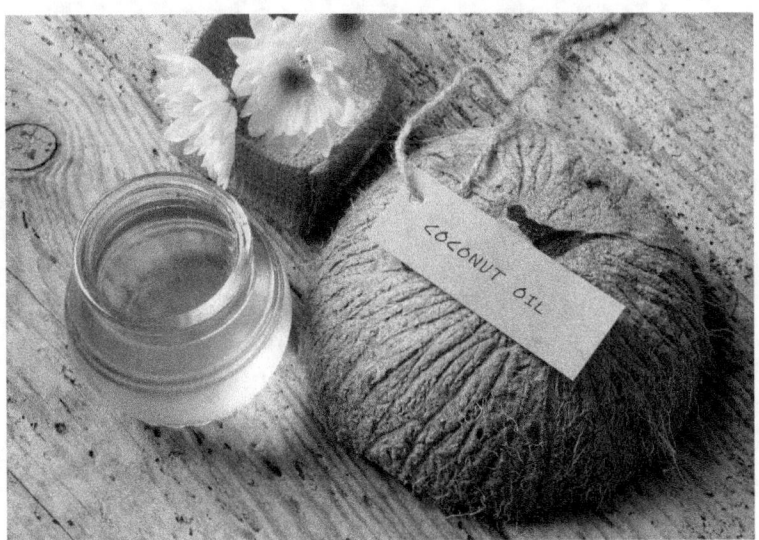

Ingredients:

- 1 cup organic coconut oil
- 1 teaspoon jojoba oil
- 4 drops essential oil (your choice)

Instructions:

1. Melt the coconut oil in a double boiler over low heat.
2. Once melted, remove from heat and whisk in the jojoba oil.
3. Allow the mixture to cool to room temperature then stir in the essential oil.
4. Beat the mixture with a hand mixer on high speed for 6 to 8 minutes until whipped.
5. Spoon the mixture into small glass jars.

Lovely Floral Bath Salts

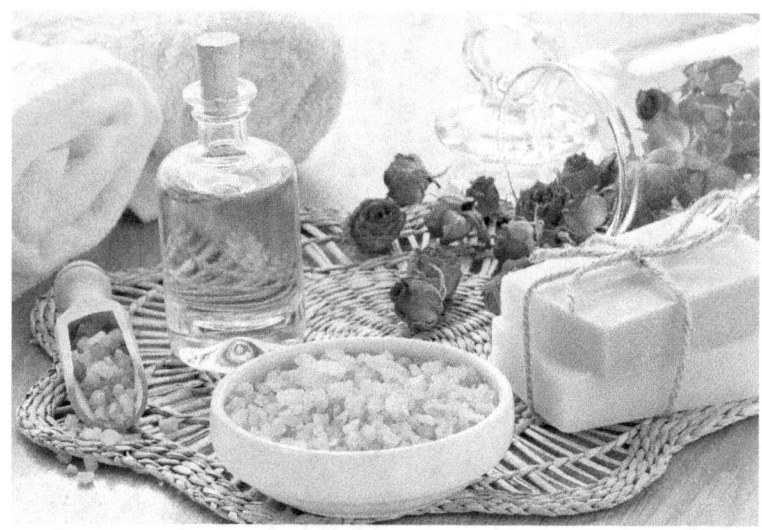

Ingredients:

- 2 cups Himalayan pink salt
- 1 tablespoon jojoba oil
- 10 drops rose essential oil
- 8 drops jasmine essential oil

Instructions:

1. Pour the salt into a mixing bowl.
2. Add the jojoba oil and essential oils.
3. Stir well to combine then pour into glass jars to store.
4. To use the salts, run a hot bath and stir in ¼ to ½ cup of salt while the water is running.
5. Stir the water by hand until the salts are dissolved.
6. Soak for at least 30 minutes then towel dry.

Invigorating Orange Lime Conditioner

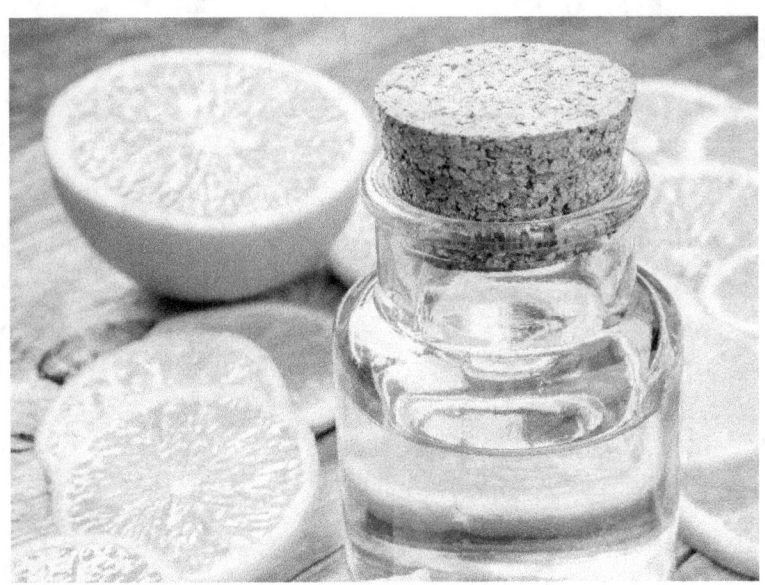

Ingredients:

- 1 cup organic coconut oil
- 1 teaspoon vitamin E oil (2 capsules)
- 1 teaspoon jojoba oil
- 4 to 6 drops orange essential oil
- 2 drops lime essential oil

Instructions:

1. Combine the coconut oil, vitamin E oil, jojoba oil and essential oils in a bowl.
2. Blend with a hand mixer until thoroughly combined.
3. Apply a small amount of the conditioner to washed hair.

4. Let it set for 3 to 5 minutes then rinse with warm water and pat dry.

Yogurt Facial Mask

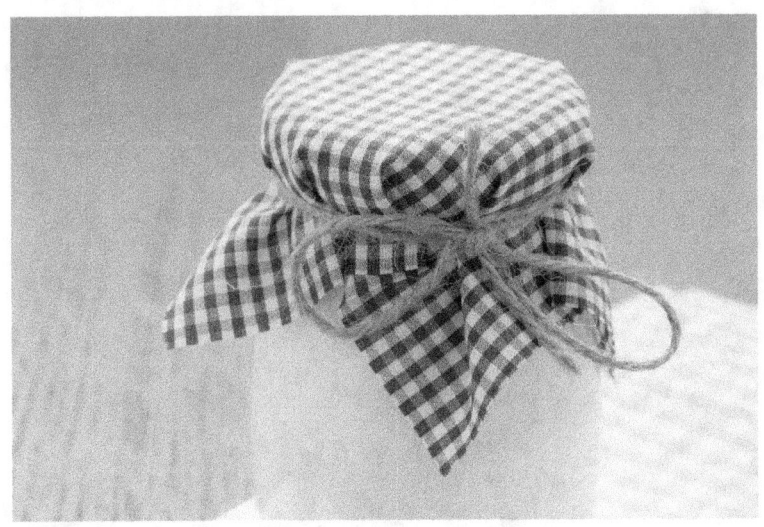

Ingredients:

- 1 slice fresh orange
- 1 tablespoon plain yogurt
- 2 teaspoons aloe
- ½ teaspoon orange zest

Instructions:

1. Squeeze the orange into a small bowl.
2. Stir in the yogurt, aloe, and orange zest.
3. Rub the mixture into the skin on your face and let rest for 5 minutes.
4. Rinse with cool water and pat dry.

Pine Fresh Shampoo

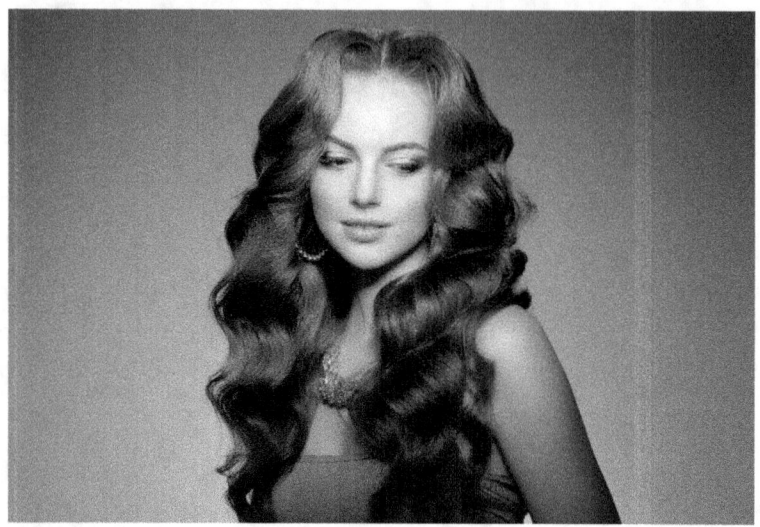

Ingredients:

- ½ cup unscented liquid castile soap
- 12 drops pine essential oil
- 4 drops cedarwood essential oil
- Filtered water, as needed

Instructions:

1. Combine the liquid soap and essential oils in an empty shampoo bottle.
2. Swirl the ingredients gently to combine.
3. Add enough water to fill the bottle the rest of the way.
4. Shake gently to combine the ingredients.
5. Apply a small amount of shampoo to damp hair and work into a lather.

6. Rinse your hair with warm water then towel dry.

Perky Peppermint Lip Balm

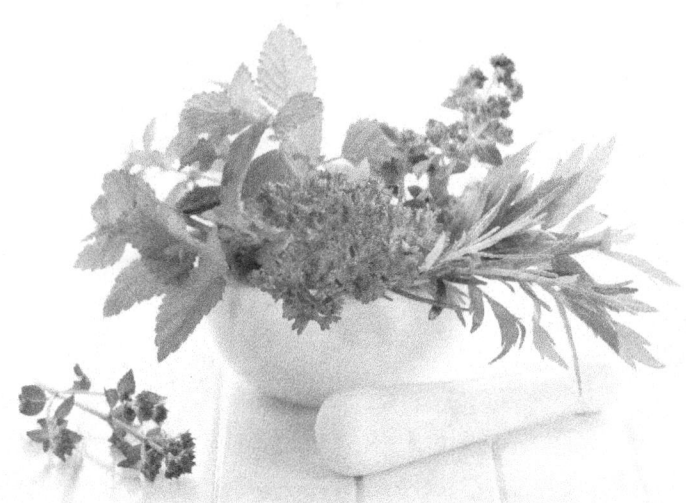

Ingredients:

- 2 tablespoons organic coconut oil
- 1 ½ tablespoons organic cocoa butter
- 1 ½ tablespoons beeswax granules
- 1 teaspoon raw honey
- 1 tablespoon jojoba oil
- 10 drops peppermint essential oil

Instructions:

1. Combine the coconut oil, cocoa butter, beeswax and honey in a double boiler over low heat.
2. Heat until the ingredients are melted then whisk smooth and remove from heat.
3. Whisk in the jojoba oil and essential oil.

4. Pour the mixture into empty lip balm tubes and let them rest upright at room temperature until solidified.

Energy-Boosting Coffee Scrub

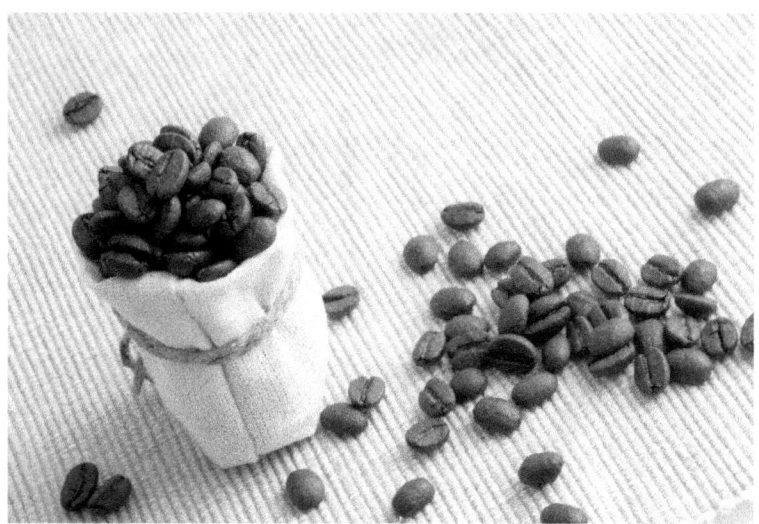

Ingredients:

- 1 cup organic coconut oil
- ½ cup organic cane sugar, coarse grain
- ¼ cup coffee grounds
- 3 tablespoons organic olive oil

Instructions:

1. Stir together the coconut oil, sugar, coffee grounds and olive oil in a mixing bowl.
2. Stir well then spoon the mixture into a glass jar.
3. Apply a small amount of the mixture to damp skin.
4. Gently scrub your face with your fingers then rinse with cool water and pat dry.

Sweet Orange Body Butter

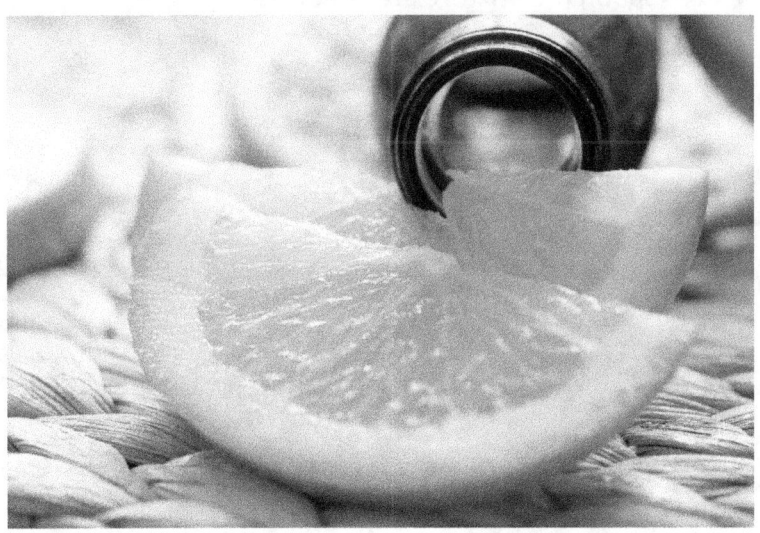

Ingredients:

- ½ cup cocoa butter
- ½ cup shea butter
- ½ cup organic coconut oil
- ½ cup sweet almond oil
- 12 drops orange essential oil

Instructions:

1. Combine the cocoa butter and shea butter in a double boiler over low heat.
2. Heat the ingredients until melted them remove from heat.
3. Whisk in the coconut oil and sweet almond oil.
4. Allow the mixture to cool to room temperature then stir in the orange essential oil.

5. Beat the mixture with a hand mixer on high speed for 6 to 8 minutes until whipped.
6. Spoon the mixture into small glass jars.

Lemon Facial Mask

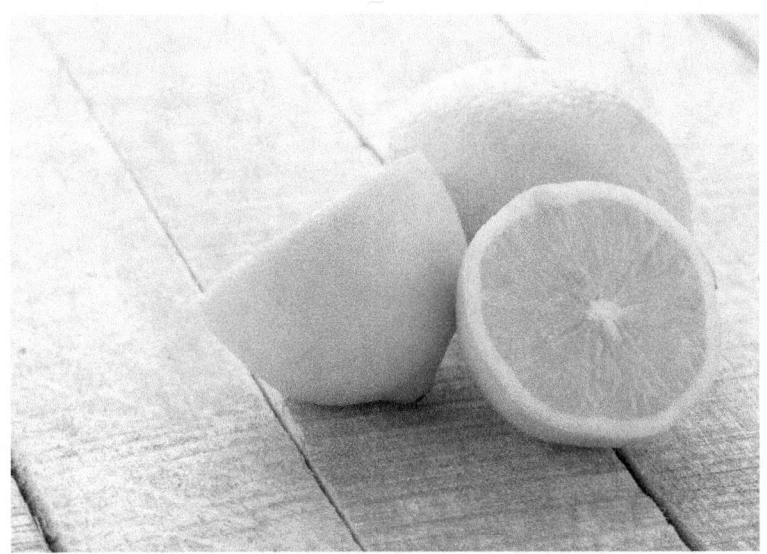

Ingredients:

- 1 ripe lemon, cut in half
- ¼ cup sweet almond oil

Instructions:

1. Squeeze the lemon into a small bowl.
2. Pour in the sweet almond oil and stir until well combined.
3. Dampen your face with warm water.
4. Apply the lemon almond oil mixture, rubbing it gently into your skin.
5. Rinse with cool water then pat your skin dry.

Conclusion

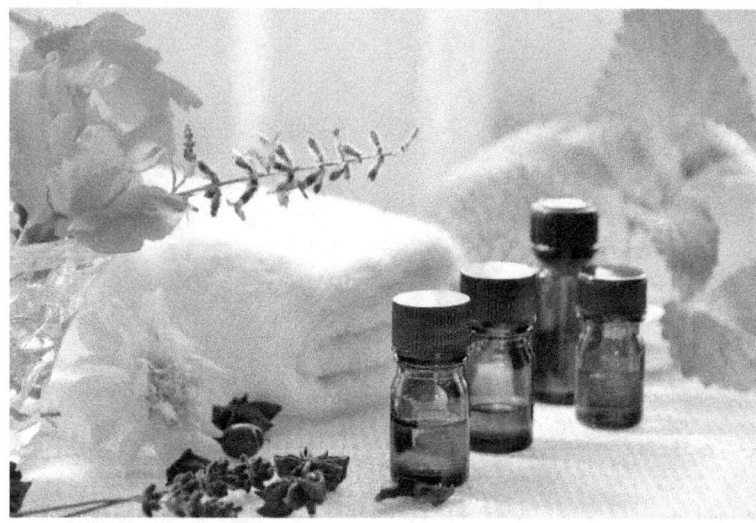

You don't have to pay a fortune for organic skin and beauty products! You can gain all the benefits of organic products without having to drain your bank account. The secret? Making your own homemade organic skin and beauty products right in your own kitchen! Making organic beauty products is easier than you might think and you can customize your recipes to suit your preferences! If you are ready to try it for yourself, just pick a recipe from this book and get going! You won't be disappointed.